ERYTHROMYCIN GUIDE TO MEN

How erythromycin can be used properly to reduce the effect of antibiotic and fungus

HILDA JOE

Table of Contents

Chapter1 3

  Mechanism of Erythromycin 3

Chapter2 13

  Precautions and Warnings of
Erythromycin 13

Chapter3 30

  Side Effects of Erythromycin 30

  The end 48

Chapter 1

Mechanism of Erythromycin

Erythromycin is a macrolide antibiotic that plays a significant role in the treatment of various bacterial infections. It operates primarily by inhibiting protein synthesis in susceptible bacteria, which disrupts their ability to grow and reproduce. Understanding the mechanism of action of erythromycin provides insights into how it effectively combats infections and the reasons behind its usage in clinical settings.

1. Structure and Pharmacokinetics

Erythromycin is derived from the fermentation products of the bacterium *Saccharopolyspora erythraea*. Its structure consists of a large lactone ring linked to one or more sugar moieties. This unique structure allows it to interact effectively with bacterial ribosomes, the cellular machinery responsible for protein synthesis.

Once administered, erythromycin can be absorbed through the gastrointestinal tract and distributed widely throughout the body. It penetrates various tissues, including the lungs, liver, and kidneys, allowing it to reach sites of infection effectively. The antibiotic is primarily excreted through bile, which is crucial for maintaining therapeutic levels, especially in treating infections of the respiratory and gastrointestinal tracts.

2. Targeting Bacterial Ribosomes

The primary action of erythromycin occurs at the ribosomal level, specifically targeting the 50S subunit of bacterial ribosomes. In bacteria, ribosomes are composed of ribosomal RNA (rRNA) and proteins. The 50S subunit, in particular, is critical for the elongation phase of protein synthesis.

When erythromycin binds to the 23S rRNA within the 50S ribosomal subunit, it effectively blocks the exit tunnel through which newly synthesized polypeptides exit the ribosome. This binding occurs at a specific site known as the peptidyl transferase center (PTC). By inhibiting this process, erythromycin prevents the addition of new amino acids to the growing polypeptide chain, leading to the premature termination of protein synthesis.

3. Inhibition of Protein Synthesis

The inhibition of protein synthesis is a crucial aspect of erythromycin's mechanism. Proteins are essential for various cellular functions, including metabolism, cell division, and structural integrity. By halting protein production, erythromycin disrupts vital processes within the bacterial cell, ultimately leading to cell death or stasis.

Erythromycin primarily exhibits bacteriostatic properties, meaning it inhibits bacterial growth and reproduction rather than directly killing the bacteria. This characteristic is particularly useful in treating infections caused by certain types of bacteria, allowing the host's immune system to eliminate the remaining pathogens. However, in high concentrations, erythromycin can exhibit bactericidal effects against some sensitive organisms.

4. Spectrum of Activity

Erythromycin is effective against a wide range of gram-positive bacteria, including *Staphylococcus* and *Streptococcus* species. Additionally, it has activity against some gram-negative bacteria, atypical pathogens, and even certain strains of *Mycoplasma* and *Chlamydia*. This broad spectrum makes erythromycin a valuable option in treating various infections, particularly respiratory tract infections, skin infections, and sexually transmitted diseases.

However, its effectiveness can be limited by bacterial resistance mechanisms. Some bacteria produce enzymes that can inactivate erythromycin, while others may alter their ribosomal target sites, reducing the antibiotic's ability to bind effectively. This has led to increased interest in alternative treatments and the development of newer antibiotics.

5. Clinical Implications and Usage

Erythromycin is commonly prescribed for patients with penicillin allergies or those who cannot tolerate beta-lactam antibiotics. Its use is especially significant in treating respiratory infections, including pneumonia, bronchitis, and sinusitis, as well as skin and soft tissue infections.

In addition to its antibacterial properties, erythromycin has anti-inflammatory effects, which can be beneficial in treating conditions like acne and certain dermatological disorders. Its ability to modulate immune responses has opened avenues for its use in combination therapies and as an adjunct treatment.

6. Considerations and Side Effects

While erythromycin is generally well-tolerated, it can cause side effects, including gastrointestinal disturbances, such as nausea, vomiting, and diarrhea. These side effects are often dose-dependent and can be managed by adjusting the dosage or using enteric-coated formulations to minimize gastrointestinal irritation.

Additionally, drug interactions can occur with erythromycin due to its effect on hepatic enzymes, particularly the cytochrome P450 system. This can lead to altered metabolism of other medications, necessitating caution when co-prescribing with other drugs.

Conclusion

In summary, erythromycin's mechanism of action is primarily centered around its ability to inhibit bacterial protein synthesis by binding to the 50S ribosomal subunit. This inhibition leads to a cessation of vital processes within the bacteria, preventing their growth and replication. Its effectiveness against various gram-positive and some gram-negative bacteria, along with its anti-inflammatory properties, makes it a versatile antibiotic. However, considerations regarding resistance, side effects, and potential drug interactions underscore the importance of appropriate clinical use and monitoring.

Chapter 2

Precautions and Warnings of Erythromycin

Erythromycin is a macrolide antibiotic widely used to treat a variety of bacterial infections. While it is generally considered safe and effective, like any medication, it carries certain risks that must be carefully managed. These risks arise from its potential side effects, drug interactions, and contraindications in specific populations. Understanding the precautions and warnings associated with erythromycin is critical for healthcare providers and patients alike to ensure its safe and effective use. This section will explore various safety concerns related to erythromycin, including its effects on different organ systems, its interactions with other medications, and special considerations for particular populations.

1. Allergic Reactions and Hypersensitivity

One of the most serious warnings associated with erythromycin is the potential for allergic reactions or hypersensitivity. Although these reactions are relatively uncommon, they can range from mild to life-threatening. Individuals who are allergic to erythromycin or other macrolide antibiotics may experience symptoms such as skin rashes, itching, or hives. In some cases, erythromycin can trigger a more severe allergic response known as anaphylaxis.

Anaphylaxis is a rapid, life-threatening condition that requires immediate medical attention. Symptoms of anaphylaxis include difficulty breathing, swelling of the throat or tongue, a rapid or irregular heartbeat, dizziness, and a drop in blood pressure. If left untreated, it can lead to loss of consciousness and even death. Due to the severity of this potential reaction, it is critical for patients with a known allergy to erythromycin or other macrolides to inform their healthcare provider before starting the medication. In the event of an allergic reaction, erythromycin should be discontinued immediately, and emergency treatment, such as administration of epinephrine, should be provided.

2. Gastrointestinal Side Effects and Risks

Erythromycin is known for causing gastrointestinal side effects, which are among the most common adverse effects associated with its use. These side effects are usually mild to moderate and include nausea, vomiting, diarrhea, abdominal pain, and cramping. Erythromycin stimulates motility in the gastrointestinal tract by acting on motilin receptors, leading to increased contractions of the stomach and intestines. While this property can be beneficial in treating conditions like gastroparesis (delayed gastric emptying), it can also cause discomfort in some individuals.

For patients with pre-existing gastrointestinal conditions, such as irritable bowel syndrome (IBS) or inflammatory bowel disease (IBD), erythromycin may exacerbate symptoms. Patients who are prone to gastrointestinal disturbances should be closely monitored when taking erythromycin, and if severe symptoms develop, alternative antibiotics may need to be considered.

A more serious gastrointestinal risk associated with erythromycin is the potential development of *pseudomembranous colitis*, a condition caused by an overgrowth of *Clostridium difficile* bacteria. This infection can lead to severe inflammation of the colon and result in symptoms such as watery diarrhea, abdominal pain, and fever. In some cases, pseudomembranous colitis can be life-threatening, and immediate discontinuation of erythromycin, along with appropriate treatment for *C. difficile* infection, is necessary.

3. Hepatic Concerns and Liver Toxicity

The liver is responsible for metabolizing erythromycin, which makes it important to consider the effects of this antibiotic on liver function. Erythromycin has been associated with cases of liver toxicity, particularly in individuals with pre-existing liver disease or those who are taking other medications that affect liver function.

One notable hepatic side effect of erythromycin is *cholestatic hepatitis*, a condition where bile flow from the liver is obstructed, leading to the buildup of bile acids in the liver and bloodstream. Symptoms of cholestatic hepatitis include jaundice (yellowing of the skin and eyes), dark urine, light-colored stools, fatigue, and abdominal pain. This condition is typically reversible once erythromycin is discontinued, but in severe cases, it may cause long-term liver damage.

Individuals with a history of liver disease, such as hepatitis, cirrhosis, or fatty liver disease, should use erythromycin with caution. Regular monitoring of liver function through blood tests is recommended for patients who require long-term erythromycin therapy or those with pre-existing liver conditions. If signs of liver dysfunction, such as elevated liver enzymes or jaundice, are observed, discontinuation of the medication and further evaluation may be necessary.

4. Cardiac Risks: QT Prolongation and Arrhythmias

Erythromycin is known to affect the electrical activity of the heart, specifically by prolonging the QT interval, which is a measurement of the time it takes for the heart's electrical system to reset between beats. Prolongation of the QT interval increases the risk of developing a potentially fatal arrhythmia called *torsades de pointes*, a type of ventricular tachycardia. This condition can lead to fainting, seizures, or even sudden death if not treated promptly.

Certain individuals are at higher risk for erythromycin-induced QT prolongation. These include individuals with a family history of long QT syndrome, patients with pre-existing heart conditions such as heart failure or bradycardia (slow heart rate), and those who are taking other medications that also prolong the QT interval. Drugs that can interact with erythromycin to increase this risk include certain antiarrhythmics, antipsychotics, antidepressants, and other macrolide antibiotics. Electrolyte imbalances, such as low potassium or magnesium levels, can further increase the risk of arrhythmias when taking erythromycin.

Patients who are at risk for QT prolongation should be evaluated before starting erythromycin, and if possible, alternative antibiotics that do not affect the heart's electrical system should be considered. In cases where erythromycin is necessary, healthcare providers may conduct regular electrocardiograms (ECGs) to monitor the QT interval and detect any early signs of arrhythmias.

5. Drug Interactions

Erythromycin is known to interact with a wide range of other medications, which can either increase the risk of side effects or reduce the effectiveness of the drugs involved. One of the primary mechanisms through which erythromycin interacts with other medications is by inhibiting certain liver enzymes, particularly the cytochrome P450 (CYP450) family, specifically the CYP3A4 enzyme. This enzyme is responsible for metabolizing many drugs, and when erythromycin inhibits it, the blood levels of other medications can increase, leading to an elevated risk of toxicity.

Anticoagulants: Erythromycin can interact with anticoagulant medications like warfarin, increasing the risk of bleeding. This is because erythromycin can inhibit the metabolism of warfarin, leading to higher concentrations in the bloodstream and an increased anticoagulant effect. Patients taking both erythromycin and anticoagulants should have their blood clotting times (INR) closely monitored to avoid the risk of excessive bleeding.

Statins: Erythromycin can also interact with cholesterol-lowering medications such as statins. By inhibiting the metabolism of statins, erythromycin can raise statin levels in the blood, increasing the risk of side women when bacterial infections need to be treated. However, certain formulations of erythromycin should be used with caution. Some studies have suggested an increased risk of adverse outcomes, such as congenital defects or miscarriage, when erythromycin is taken during pregnancy, though these risks are generally considered low.

In breastfeeding women, erythromycin can be passed to the infant through breast milk. Although this is usually safe, there is a potential risk of gastrointestinal side effects in the nursing infant, such as diarrhea or vomiting. Breastfeeding mothers should consult their healthcare provider before taking effects like muscle pain, weakness, and rhabdomyolysis (a serious condition involving muscle breakdown).

Other Antibiotics: Co-administration of erythromycin with other macrolide antibiotics or medications that prolong the QT interval can increase the risk of cardiac arrhythmias. Patients should inform their healthcare providers of all medications they are taking to avoid potentially harmful interactions.

6. Use in Pregnancy and Breastfeeding

Erythromycin is generally considered safe for use during pregnancy, and it is often prescribed to pregnant erythromycin to discuss any potential risks and whether alternative antibiotics may be more suitable.

7. Renal Impairment

Although erythromycin is primarily metabolized by the liver, a small portion of the drug is excreted through the kidneys. Patients with renal impairment or chronic kidney disease (CKD) may require dose adjustments to avoid drug accumulation in the body, which can increase the risk of toxicity. Kidney function should be monitored in patients with renal impairment who are prescribed erythromycin, and healthcare providers may need to adjust the dosage or dosing interval based on the severity of the renal dysfunction.

8. Antibiotic Resistance and Superinfections

The widespread use of antibiotics, including erythromycin, has contributed to the global issue of antibiotic resistance. Over time, bacteria can develop mechanisms to resist the effects of antibiotics, rendering them less effective. To minimize the development of resistant strains, erythromycin should be used only when necessary and prescribed by a healthcare provider for bacterial infections that are confirmed or strongly suspected to be caused by susceptible organisms.

In some cases, the use of erythromycin can lead to the development of superinfections, where resistant bacteria or fungi overgrow in response to the disruption of normal microbial flora. Patients who develop new or worsening symptoms, such as persistent fever, unusual discharge, or other signs of infection, should seek medical attention promptly, as these may indicate a superinfection requiring additional treatment.

Chapter 3

Side Effects of Erythromycin

Erythromycin is a commonly prescribed antibiotic from the macrolide class, used to treat a wide variety of bacterial infections, including respiratory infections, skin infections, and sexually transmitted infections. While it is effective in fighting bacterial infections, like all medications, erythromycin can cause a range of side effects, which can vary in intensity depending on the individual, the dosage, and the duration of treatment. Understanding the potential side effects of erythromycin is crucial for safe use and proper management of any adverse reactions.

Gastrointestinal Side Effects

One of the most common side effects associated with erythromycin is gastrointestinal discomfort. Many individuals experience some form of digestive upset when taking this antibiotic, which can include:

1. Nausea and Vomiting: Erythromycin often causes irritation to the lining of the stomach, leading to nausea. In more severe cases, this may progress to vomiting, especially when taken on an empty stomach. To minimize this side effect, it is typically recommended to take erythromycin with food. However, even when taken with

a meal, nausea and vomiting may still occur for some individuals.

2. Diarrhea: Another common side effect is diarrhea. Erythromycin works by disrupting the bacterial flora in the gut, which can sometimes lead to gastrointestinal upset. Diarrhea may range from mild to severe, and in some cases, it can lead to dehydration if not managed properly. It is essential to drink plenty of fluids and maintain hydration if this side effect occurs.

3. Abdominal Pain and Cramping: Erythromycin can cause cramping and discomfort in the

stomach and intestines. This pain may be sharp or dull and is often accompanied by bloating or a sensation of fullness. This type of abdominal discomfort is usually temporary and subsides once the body adjusts to the medication or after the completion of the treatment course.

4. Severe Diarrhea and C. difficile Infection: In more serious cases, erythromycin can disrupt the balance of bacteria in the gut to the extent that it leads to Clostridioides difficile infection (C. difficile). This bacterial infection can cause severe diarrhea, fever, abdominal pain,

and dehydration, and it requires immediate medical attention. C. difficile is a dangerous infection that can lead to colitis (inflammation of the colon) and may require a specific course of treatment to eradicate.

Allergic Reactions

As with any antibiotic, there is a possibility of an allergic reaction to erythromycin. Allergic reactions can range from mild to severe, with symptoms including:

1. Rash and Itching: Mild allergic reactions often manifest as a skin rash or itching, which may appear soon after taking the medication. This type of reaction

may be uncomfortable but is typically not dangerous unless it worsens.

2. Hives (Urticaria): Hives are raised, red, itchy welts on the skin that can vary in size. This is a more pronounced allergic reaction than a rash and may indicate a more serious response to the medication.

3. Swelling (Angioedema): Swelling, particularly around the face, lips, tongue, and throat, can occur in some individuals as a sign of an allergic reaction. This type of swelling, called angioedema, can become life-threatening if it impedes

breathing, as it may cause the airways to narrow.

4. Anaphylaxis: In rare and severe cases, erythromycin can cause anaphylaxis, a life-threatening allergic reaction. Symptoms of anaphylaxis include difficulty breathing, rapid heartbeat, swelling of the throat, severe dizziness, and loss of consciousness. Anaphylaxis requires immediate medical intervention, typically involving the administration of epinephrine and emergency care.

Skin Reactions

In addition to allergic skin reactions, erythromycin can cause various skin-related side effects. These can range from mild irritations to more severe conditions, including:

1. Photosensitivity: Erythromycin can make the skin more sensitive to sunlight, a condition known as photosensitivity. This means that individuals taking erythromycin may be more prone to sunburn, even after limited sun exposure. To avoid this, it is recommended to wear protective clothing, use sunscreen, and avoid prolonged exposure to direct sunlight while taking the medication.

2. Stevens-Johnson Syndrome (SJS) and Toxic Epidermal Necrolysis (TEN): Although rare, erythromycin has been associated with severe skin reactions, including Stevens-Johnson Syndrome (SJS) and Toxic Epidermal Necrolysis (TEN). These are serious and potentially life-threatening conditions that involve the peeling and blistering of the skin and mucous membranes. Early symptoms may include fever, sore throat, fatigue, and a red or purplish rash that spreads across the body. If SJS or TEN is suspected, erythromycin should be discontinued immediately,

and urgent medical care should be sought.

Liver-Related Side Effects

Erythromycin is metabolized in the liver, and in some cases, it can cause liver-related side effects. These can range from mild disturbances in liver function to more serious conditions such as:

1. Elevated Liver Enzymes: Erythromycin can cause an increase in liver enzyme levels, which may indicate mild liver irritation or inflammation. Elevated liver enzymes are usually detected through blood tests and may not cause noticeable symptoms. However,

if enzyme levels continue to rise or if liver function is compromised, the medication may need to be discontinued.

2. Hepatotoxicity: In more severe cases, erythromycin has been linked to liver toxicity (hepatotoxicity), which can result in liver damage. Signs of liver damage include jaundice (yellowing of the skin or eyes), dark urine, pale stools, fatigue, nausea, and abdominal pain. If any of these symptoms occur, it is essential to seek medical attention, as liver damage can become serious if not addressed promptly.

Cardiovascular Side Effects

Erythromycin can affect the heart, particularly in individuals who are predisposed to heart conditions or those taking other medications that impact heart rhythm. Some of the cardiovascular side effects include:

1. QT Prolongation: Erythromycin can cause a condition known as QT prolongation, which is an abnormality in the heart's electrical activity that can lead to arrhythmias (irregular heartbeats). QT prolongation can increase the risk of developing a potentially dangerous arrhythmia known as torsades de pointes, which can be life-threatening if not treated. Individuals with a

history of heart problems or those taking other medications that affect the heart's rhythm are at higher risk of this side effect.

2. Palpitations: Some individuals may experience heart palpitations, a sensation of the heart beating too quickly or irregularly, while taking erythromycin. While palpitations may be benign in some cases, they can also be a sign of more serious heart-related side effects, particularly in individuals with existing heart conditions.

Hearing Loss and Tinnitus

Erythromycin, particularly when taken at high doses or over extended periods, has been associated with ototoxicity, which can lead to:

1. Tinnitus: Some individuals taking erythromycin may experience tinnitus, which is a ringing or buzzing in the ears. This side effect is usually temporary and resolves once the medication is discontinued, but it can be bothersome.

2. Hearing Loss: In rare cases, erythromycin can cause hearing loss, particularly in individuals taking high doses or those with pre-existing hearing conditions. This hearing loss may be temporary or, in some cases,

permanent. It is important to report any changes in hearing to a healthcare provider immediately if this side effect occurs.

Other Common Side Effects

In addition to the more serious side effects listed above, erythromycin can cause other common and generally mild side effects, including:

1. Headaches: Mild to moderate headaches are a common side effect of erythromycin. These headaches are usually temporary and resolve on their own once the body adjusts to the medication or after the treatment course is completed.

2. Dizziness or Lightheadedness: Some individuals may experience dizziness or lightheadedness while taking erythromycin, particularly if they stand up quickly or engage in physical activity. This side effect is usually mild but should be reported if it persists or worsens.

3. Fatigue: Erythromycin can sometimes cause feelings of tiredness or fatigue, which may make individuals feel more lethargic than usual during treatment.

Precautions for Minimizing Side Effects

To minimize the risk of side effects, it is important to use erythromycin as directed by a healthcare provider. This includes taking the medication at the prescribed dosage and for the full duration of treatment, even if symptoms improve before the course is completed. Skipping doses or stopping the medication prematurely can increase the risk of bacterial resistance and may lead to the return of the infection.

Individuals with pre-existing conditions, particularly heart, liver, or kidney issues, should consult their healthcare provider before taking erythromycin, as they may be at higher risk for certain side effects. Additionally, it is crucial to inform the healthcare provider of any other medications being taken to avoid potential drug interactions.

The end

www.ingramcontent.com/pod-product-compliance
Lightning Source LLC
Chambersburg PA
CBHW030055230526
45471CB00003B/1110